World of Chillies

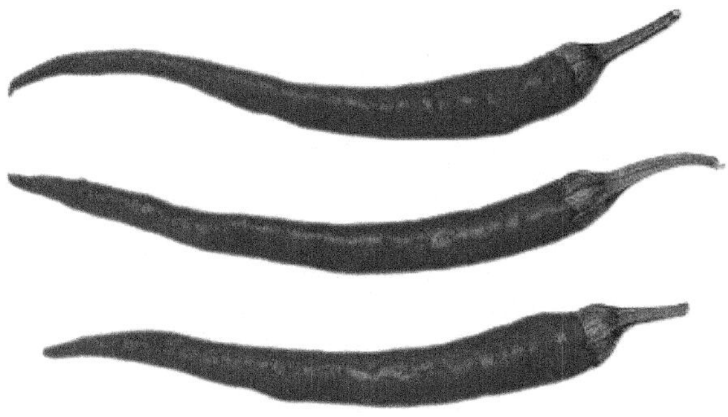

H. G. Saenger

The Book:

"World of Chillies" promises to be a comprehensive and engaging guide for anyone who wants to learn more about the tasty and versatile world of chillies. From cultivation to cooking, from health benefits to home remedies, this book offers a wealth of information to help readers appreciate and enjoy the many varieties of chillies available worldwide.

The Author:

Heinz - Günther Sänger
Passionate hobby cook
and versatile interested author,
lives since 2020 with his second
wife in Thailand

World of Chillies

"World of Chillies: Health, Taste, and Ingredients of the World's Most Flavorful Peppers"

by

H. G. Saenger

1. Edition, 2023

No.4/2 Moo.7
A.Mueang Ban Khok
67000 Phetchabun

Inhaltsverzeichnis

Table of Contents:

The Book:

In this book, „*World of Chillies: Health, Taste, and Ingredients of the World's Most Flavorful Peppers,*" the reader will embark on a journey through the fiery world of chillies. From their rich history and origins to the wide range of varieties and their Scoville heat units, this comprehensive guide will provide the reader with an appreciation for the incredible diversity of chillies worldwide.

Readers will learn about the health benefits of chillies, including the powerful effects of capsaicin, the compound responsible for their heat. The book will also explore the culinary uses of chillies, providing techniques and tips for unlocking the full potential of their flavor in the kitchen. Signature dishes from around the globe will be showcased, demonstrating the versatility and unique taste profiles of various chilli varieties.

Chilli cultivation and harvesting practices will be discussed, along with the science of heat, helping readers understand the Scoville scale and capsaicin content of their favorite peppers. To further inspire culinary creativity, the book will delve into the art of pairing chillies with other ingredients and provide guidelines for preserving and storing them.

Additionally, the book will cover chilli-based condiments and sauces, as well as home remedies and traditional uses of chillies in various cultures. To round out the reader's chilli education, the book will introduce chilli festivals and competitions that celebrate the spice and challenge the heat tolerance of participants.

„World of Chillies" promises to be a comprehensive and engaging guide for anyone interested in learning more about the flavorful and versatile world of chillies. From cultivation to cooking, health benefits to home remedies, this book will provide a wealth of information to help the reader appreciate and enjoy the many varieties of chillies available worldwide.

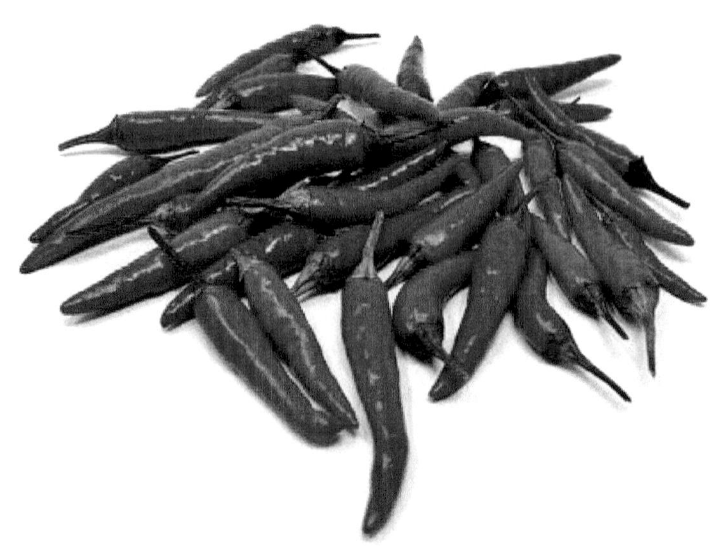

Introduction: The Fiery World of Chillies

Welcome to the fascinating and fiery world of chillies! These vibrant and flavorful peppers have captivated the hearts and palates of people around the globe for centuries, and for good reason. Ranging from mildly sweet and tangy to eye-wateringly hot, chillies offer an unmatched depth of flavor and versatility in the kitchen. In this book, „World of Chillies: Health, Taste, and Ingredients of the World's Most Flavorful Peppers," we will explore the rich history, diverse varieties, health benefits, and culinary uses of these remarkable peppers.

The story of chillies begins in the Americas, where they were first cultivated thousands of years ago. Over time, as trade routes expanded and explorers traversed the globe, chillies were introduced to other continents and quickly became a beloved ingredient in many traditional cuisines. Today, chillies are grown and consumed in almost every corner of the world, with each region boasting its own unique varieties and preparations.

As we delve into the world of chillies, we will discover the impressive range of varieties available, each with its own distinct flavor profile and heat level. We will explore the Scoville scale, which measures the heat of chillies in Scoville Heat Units (SHU), and learn about capsaicin, the compound responsible for their spiciness. From the relatively mild jala-

peno to the infamous ghost pepper, there is a chilli to suit every taste.
In addition to their culinary appeal, chillies offer a host of health benefits. Rich in vitamins and minerals, these peppers also contain capsaicin, which has been shown to have anti-inflammatory, pain-relieving, and even cancer-fighting properties. As we explore the health benefits of chillies, we will also uncover traditional home remedies and medicinal uses from various cultures around the world.

Of course, no exploration of chillies would be complete without delving into their culinary applications. We will learn how to harness the full potential of chillies in the kitchen, from techniques for controlling their heat to expert tips for pairing them with other ingredients. We will also take a journey around the globe, discovering signature dishes from various cuisines that showcase the unique flavors of different chilli varieties.

As we progress through this book, we will uncover the secrets to cultivating and harvesting chillies, as well as the science behind their heat. We will learn how to preserve and store chillies, craft fiery condiments and sauces, and even participate in chilli festivals and competitions. By the time you reach the end of this comprehensive guide, you will have gained a deep appreciation for the incredible world of chillies and the many ways they can enrich your life, both in the kitchen and beyond.

So, let's embark on this spicy journey together, and discover the vibrant, diverse, and fiery world of chillies!

The History and Origin of Chillies

The captivating journey of chillies began over 6,000 years ago in the Americas, where they were first cultivated and consumed by ancient civilizations such as the Mayans and Aztecs. Native to present-day Mexico, Central America, and parts of South America, chillies were initially used for their medicinal properties and as a means to preserve food. As time passed, they became an integral part of the culinary and cultural identity of the indigenous peoples of the Americas.

It was not until the late 15th and early 16th centuries that chillies made their way to the rest of the world. The voyage of Christopher Columbus, who set out to find a direct route to the East Indies and its valuable spices, inadvertently introduced chillies to Europe. Columbus discovered these fiery peppers in the Caribbean, mistaking them for the black pepper he sought, and brought them back to Spain.

From there, chillies quickly spread throughout Europe, Africa, and Asia, thanks to Portuguese traders who recognized their potential as a valuable commodity. As chillies were introduced to new lands, they were incorporated into local cuisines, leading to the development of countless unique dishes and flavor combinations.

One of the most significant factors in the global spread of chillies was the establishment of Portuguese and Spanish colonies in Asia. The Portuguese introduced chillies to India, where they were readily adopted into the local cuisine and eventually became a fundamental ingredient in Indian curries and spice blends. Similarly, the Spanish introduced chillies to the Philippines, which then served as a gateway to their spread throughout Southeast Asia. In each new region, the local populations embraced chillies and cultivated their own distinct varieties.

Chillies also made their way to Africa, where they were quickly adopted and integrated into traditional dishes. In West Africa, they became a key ingredient in piquant stews and sauces, while in East Africa, they were used to create fiery condiments like the popular piri-piri sauce. The African continent has since developed numerous chilli varieties, such as the Malawian Kambuzi and the Ethiopian Berbere.

Today, chillies are cultivated and consumed in virtually every corner of the world, with each region boasting its own unique varieties and preparations. The sheer diversity of chilli peppers is a testament to their adaptability and their ability to blend seamlessly into various culinary traditions. From the smoky chipotle of Mexico to the zesty bird's eye of Thailand, chillies have become an essential ingredient in countless dishes across the globe.

In summary, the history and origin of chillies can be traced back to the ancient civilizations of the Americas, where they were first cultivated and used for medicinal purposes and food preservation. Their introduction to Europe, Africa, and Asia during the Age of Exploration led to their rapid global spread and integration into numerous culinary traditions. Today, the diverse world of chillies continues to enchant and inspire cooks and food enthusiasts alike, offering an unmatched depth of flavor and versatility in the kitchen.

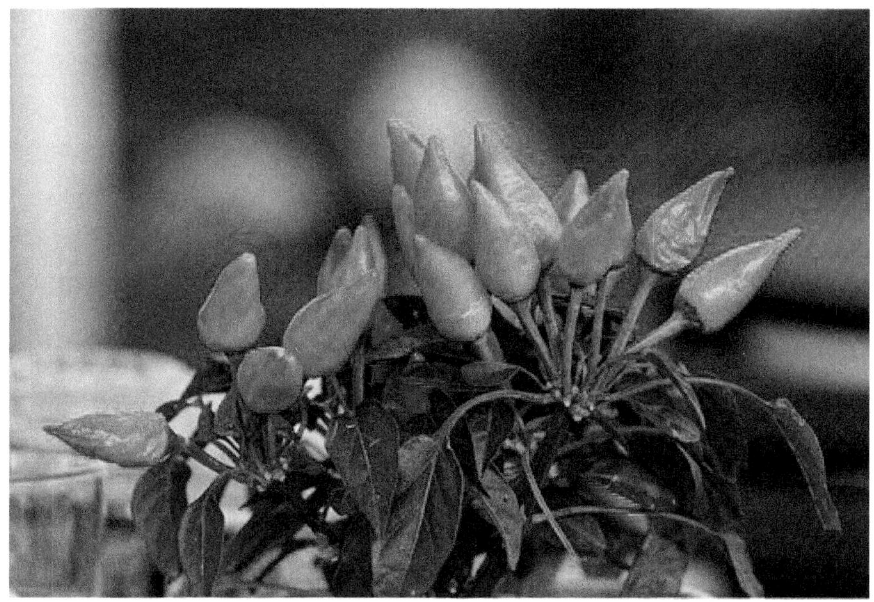

An Overview of Chilli Varieties and Their Scoville Heat Units

Chillies come in a wide range of varieties, each with its own distinct flavor profile and heat level. To help navigate this diverse world of peppers, it's useful to understand the Scoville scale, which measures the heat of chillies in Scoville Heat Units (SHU). The scale ranges from zero (no heat) to over two million (extremely hot), with the heat level of a chilli pepper determined by the amount of capsaicin it contains.

Here is an overview of some of the most popular chilli varieties and their Scoville heat units:

Jalapenos: One of the most widely recognized chilli varieties, jalapenos range from 2,500 to 8,000 SHU. They are a popular ingredient in Mexican cuisine and are often pickled or used in salsas and sauces.

Habaneros: Known for their intense heat and fruity flavor, habaneros range from 100,000 to 350,000 SHU. They are a staple in Caribbean and Latin American cuisine and are often used to make hot sauces.

Bird's Eye: A small, thin chilli commonly used in Southeast Asian cuisine, bird's eye chillies range from 50,000 to 100,000

SHU. They are often used to add heat and flavor to curries, stir-fries, and marinades.
Cayenne: A staple in Cajun and Creole cuisine, cayenne chillies range from 30,000 to 50,000 SHU. They are often used to add heat to sauces, soups, and stews.

Poblano: A mild chilli pepper often used in Mexican cuisine, poblanos range from 1,000 to 1,500 SHU. They are a popular stuffing pepper and are also used to make the traditional Mexican dish, chiles rellenos.

Thai Chilies: Commonly used in Thai cuisine, Thai chillies range from 50,000 to 100,000 SHU. They are often used to add heat to stir-fries, soups, and curries.

Ghost Peppers: One of the hottest chilli peppers in the world, ghost peppers range from 855,000 to over one million SHU. They are often used sparingly in spicy dishes and can be found in hot sauces and salsas.

In addition to these popular chilli varieties, there are countless other peppers available, each with its own unique flavor and heat profile. Whether you prefer mild peppers like bell peppers or enjoy the intense heat of a ghost pepper, there is a chilli out there to suit every taste. Understanding the Scoville scale and the heat level of each variety can help you choose the perfect chilli for your next dish.

The Health Benefits of Chillies: Capsaicin and Beyond

Chillies are not only a flavorful addition to meals but are also packed with health benefits. The active ingredient responsible for the heat in chillies is capsaicin, which has been shown to have numerous medicinal properties. Here are some of the health benefits of chillies:

Pain relief: Capsaicin has been shown to have pain-relieving properties. It works by blocking the nerve receptors that transmit pain signals to the brain, providing relief from conditions like arthritis, neuropathy, and migraines.

Anti-inflammatory: Inflammation is the root cause of many chronic diseases. Capsaicin has been shown to reduce inflammation by suppressing the production of inflammatory cytokines, which can lead to improved symptoms in conditions like asthma, allergies, and rheumatoid arthritis.

Weight loss: Capsaicin has been found to aid in weight loss by increasing metabolism and reducing appetite. Studies have shown that consuming chillies can help burn calories and reduce body fat.

Cardiovascular health: Chillies have been shown to have a positive effect on cardiovascular health by reducing blood pressure, improving circulation, and reducing the risk of heart disease.

Cancer-fighting properties: Capsaicin has been shown to have anti-cancer properties by inhibiting the growth of cancer cells and inducing apoptosis (cell death) in cancer cells. While more research is needed, chillies may have a role in cancer prevention and treatment.

Beyond capsaicin, chillies are also a rich source of vitamins and minerals, including vitamin C, vitamin A, potassium, and iron. They are also low in calories and high in fiber, making them a nutritious addition to any diet.

It's important to note that while chillies have many health benefits, they may not be suitable for everyone. People with gastrointestinal issues like ulcers or heartburn should exercise caution when consuming chillies, as they can exacerbate symptoms. Additionally, capsaicin can be irritating to the skin and eyes, so care should be taken when handling hot peppers.

In summary, chillies offer a wide range of health benefits beyond their delicious flavor. From reducing inflammation to aiding in weight loss, these fiery peppers can provide numerous benefits to your health. However, as with any food or supplement, it's important to consult with a healthcare provider before incorporating chillies into your diet.

Chillies in the Kitchen: Unlocking the Power of Flavor

Chillies are a versatile ingredient that can add a bold, complex flavor to a wide range of dishes. With so many different varieties available, each with its own distinct flavor profile and heat level, there are endless possibilities for incorporating chillies into your cooking. Here are some tips for unlocking the power of flavor in chillies in the kitchen:

Choose the right variety: Different chilli varieties have different flavors and heat levels. For example, jalapenos have a mild heat and a slightly sweet flavor, while habaneros are much hotter and have a fruity, almost tropical flavor. Experiment with different varieties to find the ones that work best for your taste preferences and the dish you're making.

Understand the heat: The heat of chillies is measured in Scoville Heat Units (SHU), with milder varieties like bell peppers having no heat and the hottest varieties like the Carolina Reaper topping out at over 2 million SHU. When cooking with chillies, it's important to understand the heat level of the variety you're using and adjust the amount accordingly.

Control the heat: If you're using a variety of chilli that is hotter than you prefer, there are several ways to control the heat. Removing the seeds and membranes, where much of the capsaicin (the compound responsible for the heat) is concentrated, can help reduce the heat level. Additionally, pairing the chillies with cooling ingredients like yogurt, sour cream, or coconut milk can help temper the heat.

Add at the right time: When cooking with chillies, it's important to add them at the right time to ensure that they don't overpower the other flavors in the dish. For example, adding chopped fresh chillies to a stir-fry at the beginning of cooking will result in a much hotter dish than adding them towards the end.

Pair with complementary flavors: Chillies pair well with a wide range of flavors, including citrus, garlic, ginger, and cilantro. Experiment with different flavor combinations to find the ones that work best for the dish you're making.

Use in a variety of dishes: Chillies can be used in a wide range of dishes, from soups and stews to sauces and marinades. They can also be used to add a kick to desserts like chocolate and ice cream.

In summary, chillies are a versatile and flavorful ingredient that can add depth and complexity to a wide range of dishes. By understanding the heat level of different varieties, controlling the heat, and pairing with complementary flavors, you can unlock the full potential of chillies in your cooking.

Exploring the Tastes and Flavors of the World's Most Popular Chillies

Chillies are used in cuisines all over the world, each with its own unique varieties and preparations. Here, we will explore some of the most popular and widely used chillies in cooking, and the distinct tastes and flavors they bring to a dish.

Jalapenos are a type of chilli pepper that are widely used in Mexican cuisine. They have a mild to medium level of heat, making them accessible to most palates, and are known for their slightly sweet and tangy flavor. Jalapenos are incredibly versatile and can be used in a variety of dishes, including salsas, sauces, and soups. They are also commonly pickled and served as a condiment, or stuffed with cheese and fried to make delicious jalapeno poppers. When selecting jalapenos, look for ones that are firm and have a vibrant green color. As they mature, they will turn red and become hotter in flavor. Whether you're using them in a traditional Mexican dish or experimenting with a new recipe, jalapenos are a great way to add flavor and a touch of heat to your cooking.

Habaneros are one of the hottest chilli peppers available, with a Scoville rating ranging from 100,000 to 350,000 units. Despite their intense heat, habaneros are also known for their unique fruity and almost floral flavor, making them a favorite in

Caribbean and Latin American cuisine. These peppers are often used to add heat and flavor to sauces, marinades, and spice rubs for grilled meats.
When using habaneros, it's important to handle them with care as they can irritate the skin and eyes. It's best to wear gloves and avoid touching your face or eyes when working with these peppers. Habaneros can be used fresh or dried, and can be added to dishes whole, sliced, or chopped. If you're sensitive to heat, use habaneros sparingly or substitute them with a milder chilli pepper. Whether you're looking to add some fiery heat to your cooking or trying to impress your guests with a bold and flavorful dish, habaneros are a great choice.

Bird's Eye chillies, also known as Thai chillies, are small but pack a mighty punch when it comes to heat. They are commonly used in Southeast Asian cuisine, particularly in Thai and Vietnamese dishes. These chillies have a distinct, fiery flavor that pairs well with coconut milk and lemongrass in curries, or added to stir-fries and noodle dishes for a spicy kick.

Bird's Eye chillies are typically green when unripe, and turn red as they mature. They can be used fresh or dried, and are often added whole or sliced to dishes for flavor and heat. When working with Bird's Eye chillies, it's important to handle them with care as they can irritate the skin and eyes. To reduce the heat level, remove the seeds and white membrane before adding them to your dish.

Bird's Eye chillies are a great way to add a bold and spicy flavor to your cooking, and are essential in many Southeast Asian dishes. If you're new to cooking with chillies or have a low tolerance for heat, start with a small amount and gradually increase as desired.

Cayenne chillies are long, thin, and usually sold in powdered form. They have a medium to high heat level and are commonly used in Cajun and Creole cuisine. The cayenne chilli has a slightly sweet and smoky flavor, which pairs well with savory dishes.

Cayenne powder is a popular spice used in many recipes, including soups, stews, and sauces. It's also a common ingredient in spice blends such as chili powder and Cajun seasoning. This versatile spice can be used to add heat to a wide range of dishes, and can be adjusted to taste depending on the desired level of spiciness.

In addition to its culinary uses, cayenne pepper is also used for its health benefits. It's believed to aid digestion, boost metabolism, and promote weight loss. Cayenne pepper is also high in vitamin C and antioxidants, making it a healthy addition to your diet.

When working with cayenne powder, it's important to use caution as it can be quite spicy. It's best to start with a small amount and adjust as needed, tasting frequently to ensure you don't overpower your dish with heat.

Overall, cayenne pepper is a versatile spice that can add a unique flavor and heat to your cooking. Whether you're making a hearty stew or a spicy sauce, cayenne is a great addition to any recipe.

Poblano chillies are a mild to medium-hot variety that is a staple in Mexican cuisine. They have a rich, earthy flavor that is slightly sweet and smoky, and they're often used in chile rellenos or roasted and added to soups and stews.

Poblano chillies are usually green in color, but they turn dark brown when fully ripened. They are a versatile chilli that can be used in many different dishes, from enchiladas and tacos to salads and sandwiches.

One of the most popular uses for poblano chillies is in chile rellenos, a traditional Mexican dish where the chillies are stuffed with cheese, meat, or beans and then battered and fried. Poblano chillies are also commonly roasted and added to soups and stews to give them a rich, smoky flavor.

In addition to their culinary uses, poblanos are also a good source of vitamin C, fiber, and antioxidants. They are believed to have anti-inflammatory properties and may help lower cholesterol levels.

When working with poblano chillies, it's important to remove the seeds and membranes to reduce the heat level, as they can be quite spicy. Roasting the chillies before use can also help enhance their flavor.

Overall, poblano chillies are a versatile and flavorful ingredient that can add depth and complexity to a wide range of dishes. Whether you're making traditional Mexican cuisine or experimenting with new flavors, poblanos are a great choice for adding mild to medium heat and earthy flavor.

Thai chilies, also known as *„bird's eye"* chilies, are a staple ingredient in Thai cuisine and are also popular in other Southeast Asian cuisines. These small but mighty chillies pack a punch, with a bright, fruity flavor and a fiery kick. Thai chilies are often used fresh, either whole or sliced, to add heat to dishes such as stir-fries, soups, and curries. They can also be dried and ground into a powder for use in spice blends and seasoning pastes. Despite their intense heat, Thai chilies are prized for their complex flavor and are often paired with other ingredients like lemongrass, ginger, and coconut milk to balance their spiciness.

Ghost peppers, also known as *Bhut Jolokia*, are some of the hottest chillies in the world, with a Scoville rating that can reach over a million SHU. Native to India, these peppers have a fruity and floral flavor with a seriously intense heat. Ghost peppers are commonly used in Indian and Southeast Asian cuisine, where they're added to chutneys, sauces, and pickles to add a fiery kick. Due to their extreme heat, ghost peppers should be used with caution and in small quantities, unless you're a true heat lover.

By exploring the tastes and flavors of different chillies, you can begin to understand how they can be used to enhance the flavor profile of a wide range of dishes. Whether you're looking for mild heat or a fiery kick, there's a chilli out there to suit your taste preferences. Experiment with different varieties in your cooking and discover the unique flavors and spice that each one brings to the table.

Chilli Cultivation and Harvesting: From Seed to Spice

Chilli cultivation is an intensive process that requires careful planning and execution. Selecting the appropriate variety of chilli is critical for a successful harvest. Depending on the intended use of the chillies, growers must consider factors such as heat level, flavor, size, and color when selecting the variety.

Once the variety has been selected, the growing conditions must be optimized to ensure healthy plant growth. Chilli plants require a warm, sunny climate and well-drained soil with a pH level of 6-7. They also require consistent watering and regular fertilization to ensure optimal growth. Some growers also use pesticides and herbicides to protect the plants from pests and diseases.

Chilli seeds can be started indoors or directly sown into the ground. Starting seeds indoors allows growers to control the growing conditions and ensure a higher germination rate. Once the seedlings have sprouted, they should be transplanted into larger containers or directly into the ground, depending on the growing method.

During the vegetative stage, chilli plants require a lot of water and nutrients to support their growth. Growers must monitor the soil moisture levels and fertilize the plants regularly to ensure optimal growth. Pruning the plants can also help promote healthy growth and increase the yield.

As the plants enter the flowering stage, they will begin to produce small, white or green flowers. These flowers will eventually give way to small, green chillies, which will grow larger and change color as they mature. It is important to wait until the chillies have reached full size and color before harvesting them to ensure optimal flavor and heat level.

Harvesting chillies requires careful attention to detail to avoid damaging the plants or the fruit. Growers can use handpicking or mechanical equipment, depending on the scale of the operation. Handpicking is the preferred method for small-scale growers, as it allows them to select only the ripest and healthiest fruit. For larger-scale operations, mechanical equipment such as harvesters or conveyors can be used to increase efficiency.

After the chillies have been harvested, they can be dried, pickled, or used fresh in a variety of dishes. Drying chillies is a popular method of preservation and can be done by hanging them in a warm, dry location until they are completely dehydrated. Pickling chillies involves soaking them in vinegar and spices, which can enhance their flavor and extend their shelf life. Fresh chillies can be used in a variety of dishes, from soups and stews to salsas and curries.

In conclusion, chilli cultivation and harvesting require a lot of attention to detail and a thorough understanding of the growing conditions that are necessary for a successful harvest. By selecting the appropriate variety, providing the necessary growing conditions, and harvesting the fruit at the right time, growers can produce high-quality chillies that are perfect for a variety of culinary applications.

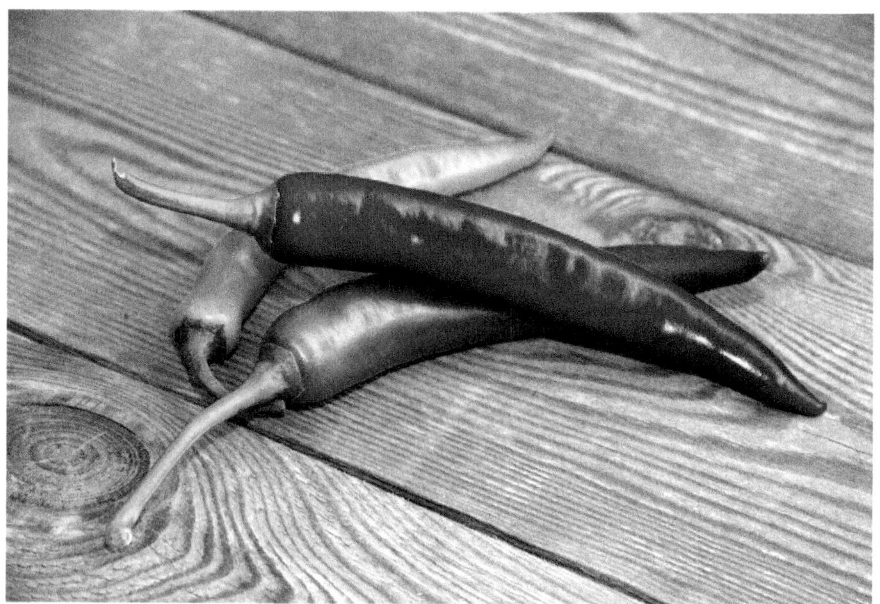

The Science of Heat: Understanding Scoville Units and Capsaicin Content.

Capsaicin is the chemical compound responsible for the pungent, fiery flavor of chili peppers. It is a natural alkaloid and belongs to the class of compounds called capsaicinoids, which are primarily found in the fruit of plants in the Capsicum genus. Capsaicin is the most abundant capsaicinoid in chili peppers, and it is responsible for the vast majority of their heat.

The intensity of the heat in chili peppers is measured using a scale known as the Scoville scale. This scale is named after its inventor, Wilbur Scoville, who developed it in 1912. The Scoville scale measures the amount of capsaicin present in a chili pepper, and it is expressed in Scoville heat units (SHU).

The Scoville scale ranges from 0 SHU for sweet peppers to over 2 million SHU for the hottest chili peppers, such as the Carolina Reaper. To determine the Scoville rating of a chili pepper, a sample is extracted with a solvent such as alcohol or water, and the extract is then diluted in sugar water until the heat is no longer detectable by a panel of taste testers. The Scoville rating is then calculated based on the degree of dilution required to eliminate the heat.

While the Scoville scale is a useful tool for measuring the heat of chili peppers, it has some limitations. One of the main limitations is that it relies on human taste testers, which can introduce subjective variability. Additionally, the Scoville scale does not take into account the presence of other capsaicinoids in chili peppers, such as dihydrocapsaicin and nordihydrocapsaicin.

To address these limitations, a more precise method of measuring capsaicin content in chili peppers was developed in the 1980s. This method, known as high-performance liquid chromatography (HPLC), separates the individual capsaicinoids in a chili pepper extract and quantifies their content based on their absorption of light at specific wavelengths. HPLC is a more objective and precise method for measuring capsaicin content than the Scoville scale.

Despite its fiery flavor, capsaicin has a range of health benefits. Studies have shown that capsaicin can boost metabolism, reduce appetite, and promote weight loss. It can also help reduce inflammation and pain, making it a potentially useful treatment for conditions such as arthritis and neuropathic pain. Additionally, capsaicin has antimicrobial properties and may help to prevent the growth of bacteria and fungi.

In conclusion, capsaicin is the compound responsible for the heat in chili peppers, and its intensity is measured using the Scoville scale or HPLC. While the Scoville scale is a useful tool for measuring the heat of chili peppers, it has some limitations, and HPLC is a more precise method. Capsaicin has a range of potential health benefits, including boosting metabolism, reducing inflammation and pain, and inhibiting the growth of bacteria and fungi.

The Art of Cooking with Chillies: Techniques and Tips

Cooking with chillies is an art that requires careful consideration of their unique flavor profiles and heat levels. Whether you're a seasoned chef or a novice in the kitchen, there are a few key techniques and tips to keep in mind when working with chillies to create delicious and flavorful dishes.
Use the Right Chilli Variety

The first step to cooking with chillies is to choose the right variety for your recipe. As discussed earlier, there are many different types of chillies, each with its own unique flavor profile and heat level. Depending on the dish you are preparing, you may want to use a mild chilli, such as the poblano, or a hotter variety, such as the habanero or ghost pepper. It's important to keep in mind that the heat level of a chilli can vary depending on factors such as growing conditions and ripeness, so it's a good idea to taste a small piece of the chilli before adding it to your recipe.

Handle with Care
When working with chillies, it's important to handle them with care to avoid irritation to your skin and eyes. Some varieties of chillies, such as the habanero and ghost pepper, can cause intense burning and even blistering if they come into contact with your skin or eyes. It's recommended to wear gloves when handling these hot peppers, and to avoid touching your face or eyes while working with them. If you do come into contact with

a hot pepper, wash your hands thoroughly with soap and water.

Balance the Heat

When adding chillies to your dish, it's important to balance the heat level with other flavors to create a well-rounded and enjoyable dish. For example, adding a sweet element such as honey or sugar can help to balance out the heat of a hot pepper, while the creaminess of coconut milk can help to mellow out the spiciness of a curry. It's also important to consider the overall flavor profile of the dish and to use chillies that complement the other ingredients.

Use the Whole Chilli

To get the most flavor out of your chillies, it's often best to use the whole pepper, including the seeds and membranes. The seeds and membranes are where most of the capsaicin, the compound responsible for the heat in chillies, is located, so removing them will reduce the overall heat level of the dish. However, if you prefer a milder dish, you can remove the seeds and membranes before using the chilli.

Cook the Chillies

Cooking chillies can help to mellow out their heat and bring out their flavor. Roasting or grilling chillies can help to give them a smoky flavor, while sautéing them in oil can help to release their flavor into the dish. It's important to keep in mind that cooking can also increase the heat level of some chillies, so be sure to taste as you go to ensure that the dish has the right level of spiciness.

Pair with Complementary Flavors

When cooking with chillies, it's important to pair them with complementary flavors to create a well-rounded dish. For example, the bright and tangy flavor of lime juice can help to balance out the heat of a spicy dish, while the earthiness of cumin can help to enhance the flavor of chillies in a Mexican-inspired dish. Experimenting with different flavor combinations can help to take your dishes to the next level.

In conclusion, cooking with chillies requires careful consideration of their unique flavor profiles and heat levels. By choosing the right variety, handling them with care, balancing the heat, using the whole pepper, cooking them properly, and pairing them with complementary flavors, you can create delicious and flavorful dishes that will impress your guests and.

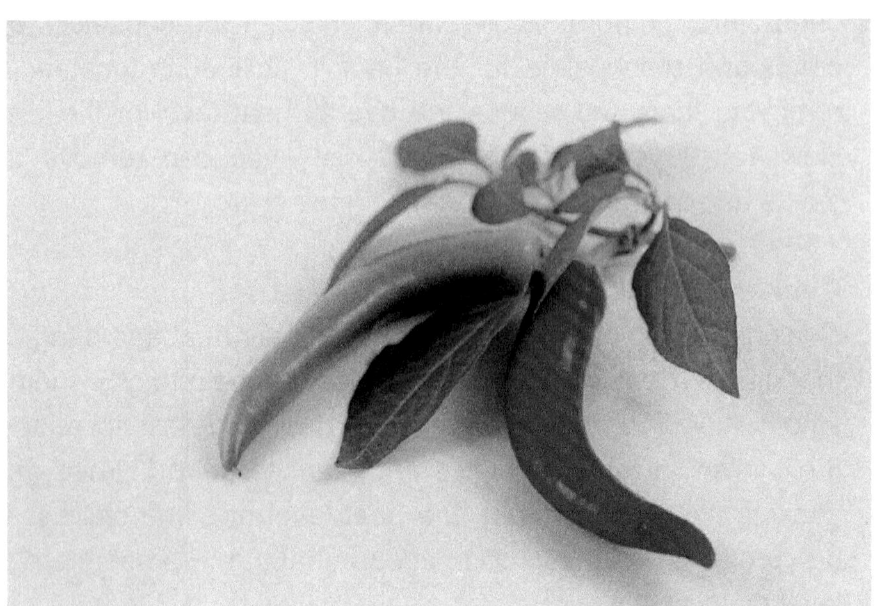

World Chilli Cuisine: Signature Dishes from Around the Globe

Chillies are used in cuisine around the world, adding heat, flavor, and color to dishes. In this chapter, we will explore some signature chilli dishes from different regions of the world.

Mexican Cuisine - Chile Relleno: A classic Mexican dish consisting of roasted poblano chillies stuffed with cheese, meat, or vegetables, then dipped in egg batter and fried. The dish is typically served with a tomato-based sauce.

Indian Cuisine - Vindaloo: Originating from the Goa region of India, Vindaloo is a fiery dish made with a blend of spices, vinegar, and red chillies. It is often made with meat, such as pork or lamb, and served with rice or naan bread.

Thai Cuisine - Tom Yum Soup: A spicy and sour soup made with lemongrass, galangal, kaffir lime leaves, and bird's eye chillies. The soup can be made with shrimp, chicken, or tofu and is typically served with rice.

Korean Cuisine - Kimchi: A traditional Korean side dish made from fermented vegetables, including cabbage, radish, and scallions, seasoned with a blend of spices, including Korean chili powder. Kimchi can be eaten on its own or used as a condiment.

Caribbean Cuisine - Jerk Chicken: A popular dish in the Caribbean, Jerk Chicken is marinated in a mixture of herbs, spices, and Scotch bonnet peppers before being grilled or smoked. The dish is typically served with rice and beans or fried plantains.

Hungarian Cuisine - Goulash: A traditional Hungarian stew made with beef or pork, onions, tomatoes, and a blend of spices, including paprika. The dish can be made with varying levels of spiciness, depending on the amount of chili used.

Chinese Cuisine - Kung Pao Chicken: A spicy stir-fry dish made with chicken, peanuts, vegetables, and Sichuan peppercorns. The dish is known for its signature heat and numbing sensation from the Sichuan peppercorns.

Ethiopian Cuisine - Doro Wat: A spicy Ethiopian stew made with chicken, onions, tomatoes, and berbere spice blend, which includes chili peppers, ginger, and other spices. The dish is typically served with injera, a spongy flatbread.

The full recipes follow on the next pages.

In conclusion, chillies are a versatile ingredient that can be found in cuisine from all over the world, adding heat and flavor to dishes. From Mexican chile rellenos to Ethiopian Doro Wat, there are countless signature dishes that showcase the unique flavors of chillies in different regions of the world.

Mexican Chile Relleno Recipe

Ingredients:

4 large poblano chillies

1 cup of grated cheese (Monterey Jack, Oaxaca or Chihuahua cheese)

1 cup of cooked ground beef or shredded chicken (optional)

1/2 cup of all-purpose flour

1/2 teaspoon of salt

4 eggs, separated

1/2 cup of vegetable oil

1 cup of tomato sauce

Instructions:

- Roast the poblano chillies over an open flame or under the broiler until the skin is charred and blistered.
- Transfer the roasted chillies to a plastic bag and let them steam for 10 minutes. This will make it easier to remove the skin.
- Carefully peel the skin off the chillies, making sure not to tear them.
- Cut a small slit in each chilli and remove the seeds and veins.
- Stuff the chillies with grated cheese and cooked meat or vegetables, if using.
- In a bowl, mix together the flour and salt. In a separate bowl, beat the egg whites until stiff peaks form. In another bowl, beat the egg yolks until they are pale yellow.
- Gently fold the beaten egg yolks into the egg whites.

- Heat the vegetable oil in a large skillet over medium-high heat.
- Dip each stuffed chilli into the flour mixture, then coat it in the egg mixture.
- Fry the coated chillies in the hot oil, turning them occasionally, until they are golden brown on all sides.
- Remove the chillies from the skillet and place them on paper towels to drain off any excess oil.
- Serve the Chile Rellenos with warm tomato sauce on top. Enjoy!

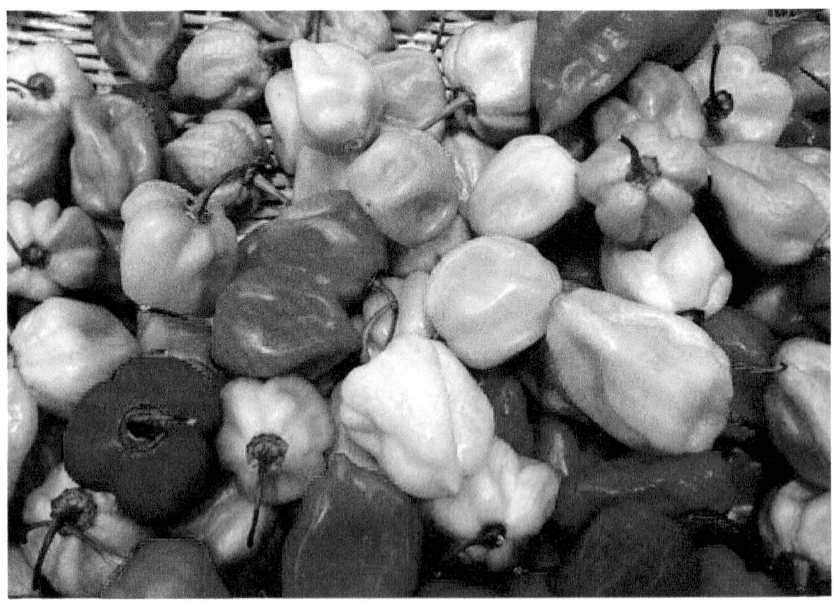

Vindaloo Recipe:

Ingredients:

1 lb. of pork or lamb, cut into cubes
1 large onion, diced
4 cloves of garlic, minced
1 tbsp. of ginger paste
2-3 fresh green chillies, chopped
1 tsp. of cumin seeds
1 tsp. of coriander seeds
1 tsp. of mustard seeds
1 tsp. of fenugreek seeds
1 tsp. of turmeric powder
1 tsp. of paprika
1 tsp. of red chilli powder
1 tbsp. of tomato paste
2 tbsp. of white wine vinegar
2 tbsp. of vegetable oil
Salt to taste

Instructions:

- In a dry pan, roast the cumin, coriander, mustard, and fenugreek seeds until fragrant. Grind the spices in a mortar and pestle or spice grinder.
- In a large pot, heat the vegetable oil over medium-high heat. Add the diced onions and sauté until translucent.

- Add the minced garlic, ginger paste, and chopped green chillies to the pot. Sauté for another minute.
- Add the ground spices, turmeric powder, paprika, and red chilli powder to the pot. Stir to combine and cook for 1-2 minutes.
- Add the tomato paste and white wine vinegar to the pot. Stir well and cook for another minute.
- Add the cubed meat to the pot and stir to coat with the spice mixture. Cook for a few minutes until the meat is browned on all sides.
- Add enough water to the pot to cover the meat. Bring to a boil and then reduce the heat to low. Cover the pot and let simmer for 45-60 minutes, or until the meat is tender.
- Add salt to taste and adjust the spices as needed. Serve hot with rice or naan bread.

Note: This recipe can be made with other meats, such as chicken or beef, or with vegetables for a vegetarian option. The spice level can also be adjusted to taste by increasing or decreasing the amount of red chilli powder used.

Here is a recipe for Tom Yum Soup:

Ingredients:

2 stalks lemongrass, cut into 2-inch pieces
4 kaffir lime leaves
2-inch piece of galangal, sliced
3-4 bird's eye chillies, finely chopped
4 cups chicken or vegetable broth
1 cup sliced mushrooms
1/2 pound shrimp, peeled and deveined
1 tablespoon fish sauce
1 tablespoon lime juice
1/4 cup chopped cilantro

Instructions:

- In a large pot, bring the broth to a boil.
- Add the lemongrass, kaffir lime leaves, galangal, and bird's eye chillies to the broth. Simmer for 5 minutes to allow the flavors to infuse.
- Add the mushrooms to the pot and simmer for another 5 minutes.
- Add the shrimp to the pot and cook for 2-3 minutes until pink.
- Add the fish sauce and lime juice to the pot and stir to combine.
- Remove the pot from the heat and stir in the chopped cilantro.

- Serve the soup hot with steamed rice.
- Enjoy the spicy and sour flavors of this classic Thai soup!

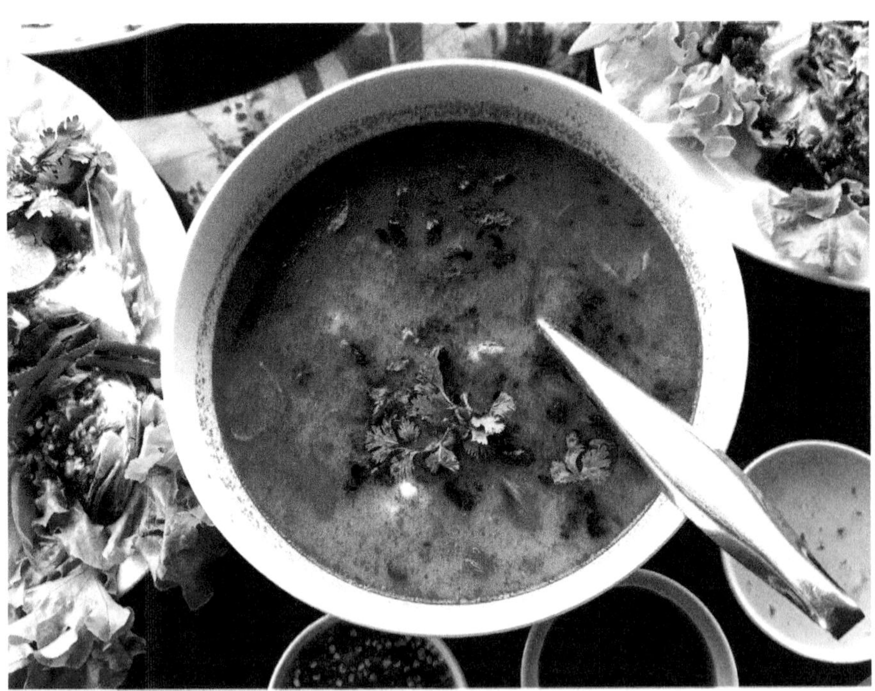

Korean Cuisine - Kimchi

Korean Cuisine - Kimchi: A traditional Korean side dish made from fermented vegetables, including cabbage, radish, and scallions, seasoned with a blend of spices, including Korean chili powder. Kimchi can be eaten on its own or used as a condiment.

Ingredients:

1 medium Napa cabbage
1/4 cup kosher salt
8 oz daikon radish, peeled and grated
4 scallions, thinly sliced
1/4 cup Korean chili powder
2 tbsp fish sauce
2 tbsp soy sauce
1 tbsp grated fresh ginger
5 cloves garlic, minced
1 tbsp sugar

Instructions:

- Cut the cabbage into quarters lengthwise and remove the core. Cut each quarter crosswise into 2-inch pieces.
- In a large bowl, mix the cabbage with the kosher salt. Let stand for 2 hours, stirring occasionally.
- Rinse the cabbage under cold water and drain well.

- In a separate bowl, mix together the daikon radish, scallions, Korean chili powder, fish sauce, soy sauce, ginger, garlic, and sugar.
- Add the cabbage to the mixture and mix well, making sure the cabbage is fully coated.
- Pack the mixture into a clean jar, pressing down firmly to remove any air bubbles.
- Cover the jar with a lid and let it sit at room temperature for 1-5 days, depending on the desired level of fermentation.
- Once the kimchi has fermented to your liking, store it in the refrigerator. It will keep for several months.

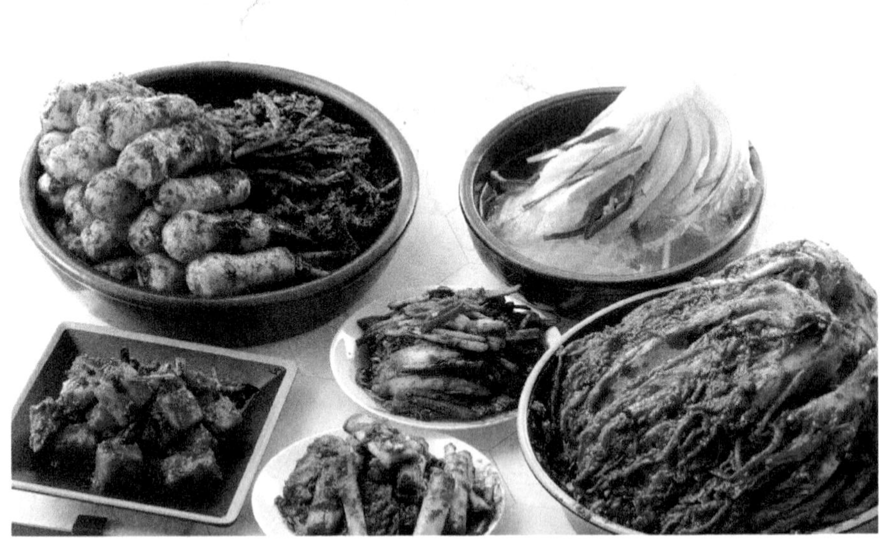

Caribbean Cuisine - Jerk Chicken

Caribbean Cuisine - Jerk Chicken: A popular dish in the Caribbean, Jerk Chicken is marinated in a mixture of herbs, spices, and Scotch bonnet peppers before being grilled or smoked. The dish is typically served with rice and beans or fried plantains.

Ingredients:

2 lbs. bone-in chicken pieces
1 onion, chopped
4 garlic cloves, minced
4-6 Scotch bonnet peppers, seeded and chopped
1 tbsp. ground allspice
1 tbsp. dried thyme
2 tsp. ground cinnamon
2 tsp. ground nutmeg
2 tbsp. brown sugar
2 tbsp. soy sauce
1 tbsp. vegetable oil
Salt and pepper to taste

Instructions:

- In a blender or food processor, combine the onion, garlic, Scotch bonnet peppers, allspice, thyme, cinnamon, nutmeg, brown sugar, soy sauce, vegetable oil, salt, and pepper. Process until smooth.
- Place the chicken pieces in a large bowl and pour the marinade over them, making sure that each piece is fully coated. Cover the bowl with plastic wrap and refrigerate for at least 2 hours, or overnight for best results.
- Preheat your grill to medium-high heat. Remove the chicken from the marinade and shake off any excess. Discard the remaining marinade.
- Grill the chicken pieces for 6-8 minutes per side, or until fully cooked and the internal temperature reaches 165°F (75°C). Serve hot with rice and beans or fried plantains.
- Note: If you don't have a grill, you can also bake the chicken in the oven at 400°F (200°C) for 30-40 minutes, or until fully cooked.

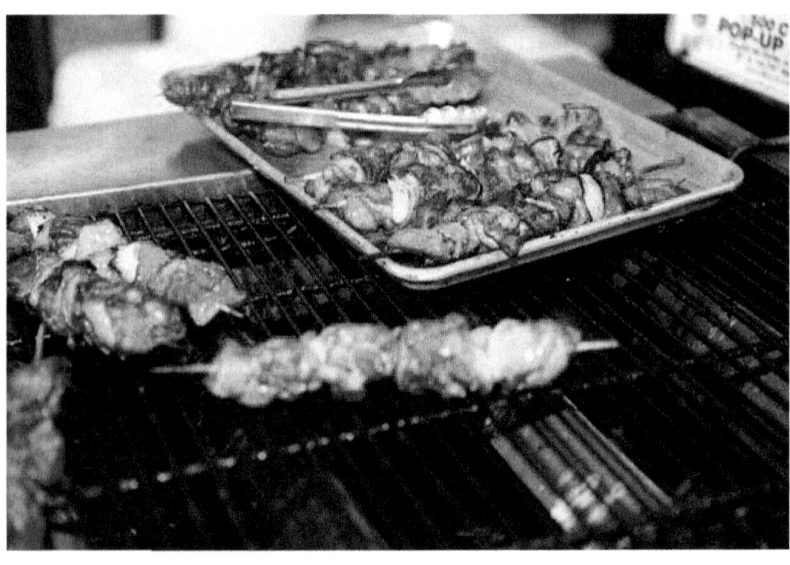

Hungarian Goulash:

Ingredients:

2 pounds of beef chuck, cut into 1-inch cubes
2 onions, chopped
2 tablespoons of vegetable oil
3 garlic cloves, minced
2 tablespoons of paprika
1 teaspoon of caraway seeds
1 teaspoon of dried marjoram
1 teaspoon of dried thyme
1 bay leaf
2 cups of beef broth
2 cups of diced tomatoes
2 green bell peppers, chopped
2 red bell peppers, chopped
Salt and black pepper to taste

Instructions:

- In a large Dutch oven, heat the vegetable oil over medium-high heat. Add the beef cubes and cook until browned on all sides, about 5 minutes. Remove the beef from the pot and set aside.
- Add the onions to the pot and cook until softened, about 5 minutes. Add the garlic, paprika, caraway seeds, marjoram, thyme, and bay leaf and cook for another 2-3 minutes, stirring constantly.

- Add the beef broth and diced tomatoes to the pot and bring to a simmer. Return the beef to the pot and stir to combine. Cover the pot and simmer for 1 hour, stirring occasionally.
- Add the chopped bell peppers to the pot and continue simmering for another 30 minutes, or until the beef is tender and the vegetables are soft. Season with salt and black pepper to taste.
- Serve the goulash hot with crusty bread or over egg noodles.
- Note: For a spicier goulash, you can add a pinch of cayenne pepper or red pepper flakes along with the paprika.

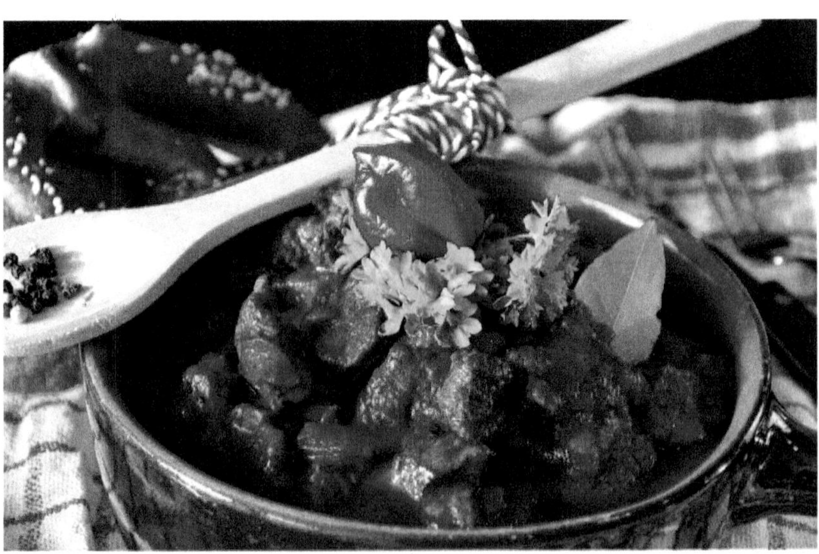

Chinese Cuisine - Kung Pao Chicken

Chinese Cuisine - Kung Pao Chicken: A spicy stir-fry dish made with chicken, peanuts, vegetables, and Sichuan peppercorns. The dish is known for its signature heat and numbing sensation from the Sichuan peppercorns.

Ingredients:

500g boneless, skinless chicken breasts, cut into small pieces
1 cup roasted peanuts
1 red bell pepper, diced
1 green bell pepper, diced
3-4 dried red chili peppers
3 cloves garlic, minced
1-inch piece of ginger, grated
2 tbsp soy sauce
2 tbsp rice vinegar
2 tbsp hoisin sauce
1 tbsp cornstarch
1 tbsp sugar
1 tsp Sichuan peppercorns
2 tbsp vegetable oil
Green onions, thinly sliced, for garnish

Instructions:

- In a small bowl, whisk together soy sauce, rice vinegar, hoisin sauce, cornstarch, sugar, and 1/4 cup of water until well combined. Set aside.
- Heat a wok or large skillet over high heat. Add vegetable oil and swirl to coat the pan.
- Add chicken and stir-fry for 2-3 minutes, until browned on all sides.
- Add dried chili peppers, garlic, and ginger, and stir-fry for 30 seconds.
- Add red and green bell peppers, and stir-fry for another 2-3 minutes, until vegetables are tender-crisp.
- Add the soy sauce mixture to the pan and stir-fry for 1-2 minutes, until the sauce thickens and coats the chicken and vegetables.
- Crush the Sichuan peppercorns using a mortar and pestle or a spice grinder.
- Add the crushed Sichuan peppercorns and roasted peanuts to the pan, and stir to combine.
- Serve hot, garnished with sliced green onions.
- Note: For a milder version, reduce the number of dried chili peppers used.

Ethiopian Cuisine - Doro Wat

Ingredients:

2 lbs chicken, cut into pieces
2 large onions, finely chopped
4 cloves garlic, minced
1-inch piece ginger, peeled and minced
3 tbsp berbere spice blend
1 tbsp paprika
1 tsp cumin
1 tsp turmeric
1 tsp salt
1 cup chicken broth
2 tbsp butter or oil
Hard-boiled eggs (optional)
Injera (for serving)

Instructions:

- In a large pot or Dutch oven, heat the butter or oil over medium-high heat. Add the onions and sauté until golden brown, about 10 minutes.
- Add the garlic and ginger and cook for an additional 2-3 minutes, until fragrant.
- Add the berbere spice blend, paprika, cumin, turmeric, and salt, and cook for another 2-3 minutes, stirring constantly.

- Add the chicken pieces to the pot and stir until they are coated in the spice mixture.
- Add the chicken broth and bring to a simmer. Reduce heat to low and cover the pot with a lid. Allow the stew to simmer for 45-60 minutes, or until the chicken is tender and cooked through.
- If desired, add hard-boiled eggs to the stew during the last 10 minutes of cooking.
- Serve the Doro Wat hot with injera, a traditional spongy flatbread used to scoop up the stew.
- Note: Berbere spice blend can be purchased at specialty stores or online, or you can make your own by combining chili powder, paprika, cumin, coriander, ginger, cardamom, cinnamon, cloves, and nutmeg.

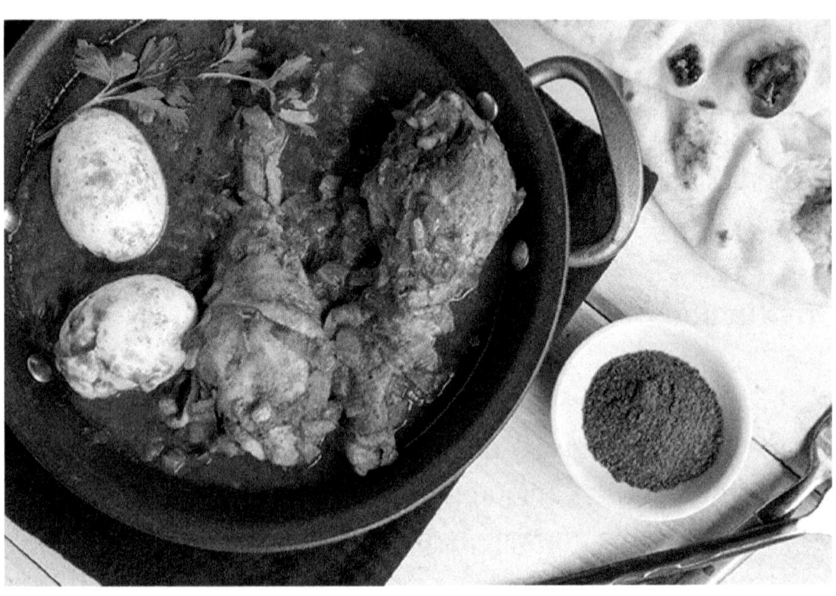

Heat and Flavor Pairings: Chilli and Ingredient Combinations

Heat and flavor pairings are essential to creating delicious dishes that balance the intensity of chillies with complementary ingredients. The following are some popular chili and ingredient combinations that work well together.

Citrus: The acidic tang of citrus fruits such as lime and lemon can help to balance out the heat of chillies, making them a perfect pairing. For example, adding a squeeze of lime to a spicy Thai curry can enhance the flavors and make the heat more tolerable.

Creamy dairy: Creamy dairy products such as yogurt, sour cream, and cheese can help to cool down the heat of spicy dishes while adding a rich, luxurious texture. For example, a dollop of sour cream on top of a spicy bowl of chili can help to balance out the heat.

Chocolate: Chocolate and chillies may seem like an unusual pairing, but the bitterness of dark chocolate can complement the heat of spicy dishes. For example, adding a square of dark chocolate to a spicy mole sauce can deepen the flavors and add complexity.

Sweet fruits: Sweet fruits such as mango, pineapple, and papaya can help to balance out the heat of spicy dishes while adding a refreshing burst of sweetness. For example, adding diced mango to a spicy salsa can add a tropical twist and help to cool down the heat.

Smoky flavors: Smoky flavors such as chipotle peppers, smoked paprika, and grilled meats can complement the heat of spicy dishes while adding depth and complexity. For example, using smoked paprika in a spicy chorizo and potato stew can add a smoky dimension to the dish.

Garlic and onions: Garlic and onions are staple ingredients in many spicy dishes, and for good reason. These pungent ingredients can help to balance out the heat while adding depth and flavor. For example, sautéing garlic and onions before adding chili powder to a dish can help to develop the flavors and make the dish more well-rounded.

In conclusion, heat and flavor pairings are crucial when cooking with chillies. By experimenting with complementary ingredients and flavors, you can create delicious dishes that balance the intensity of chili heat with other delicious and complementary flavors.

Preserving and Storing Chillies: Drying, Pickling, and More

Preserving and storing chillies is a great way to extend their shelf life and ensure that you have a supply of your favorite varieties all year round. There are several methods for preserving and storing chillies, including drying, pickling, freezing, and canning.

Drying chillies is a popular method of preservation and can be done easily at home. Simply wash and dry the chillies, then string them up by their stems and hang them in a warm, dry location until they are completely dehydrated. Once dried, they can be stored in airtight containers for later use. Dried chillies can be used in a variety of dishes, including soups, stews, and sauces, to add flavor and heat.

Pickling chillies is another popular method of preservation that can enhance their flavor and extend their shelf life. To pickle chillies, first wash and dry them, then pack them into sterilized jars. Heat vinegar, water, salt, and any desired spices in a saucepan until the salt dissolves. Pour the hot liquid over the chillies in the jars, making sure they are completely covered. Seal the jars and store in a cool, dark place for several weeks before using. Pickled chillies are great for adding to sandwiches, salads, and even cocktails.

Freezing chillies is another option for preserving them, but it is important to note that freezing can change the texture of the chillies. To freeze chillies, simply wash and dry them, then place them in airtight containers or freezer bags. They can be stored in the freezer for up to six months. Frozen chillies are best used in cooked dishes, as they may become mushy when thawed.

Canning chillies is a more advanced method of preservation that requires specific equipment and techniques. To can chillies, first wash and dry them, then pack them into sterilized jars. Heat a solution of vinegar, water, and salt in a large pot, then pour the hot liquid over the chillies in the jars, making sure they are completely covered. Seal the jars and process them in a boiling water bath for the recommended time based on your altitude and the recipe you are following. Canned chillies can be stored in a cool, dark place for up to one year.

In conclusion, there are several methods for preserving and storing chillies, including drying, pickling, freezing, and canning. Each method has its own advantages and disadvantages, and the choice of which method to use will depend on personal preference, available equipment, and the desired use of the chillies. Properly preserved and stored chillies can add flavor and heat to a variety of dishes throughout the year.

Chilli-Based Condiments and Sauces: Crafting Fiery Creations

Chilli-based condiments and sauces are popular additions to many dishes, adding flavor, heat, and complexity to meals. These sauces can be used as dips, marinades, or as a finishing touch to dishes. In this chapter, we will explore the world of chilli-based condiments and sauces and how to make them at home.

One of the most popular chilli-based condiments is hot sauce. Hot sauce can be made with a variety of chillies and ingredients, depending on personal taste preferences. To make a basic hot sauce, you will need to puree chillies with vinegar and salt, and then simmer the mixture on the stove for a few minutes. This will help to blend the flavors and create a smooth consistency. You can also add other ingredients such as garlic, onions, and spices to enhance the flavor of the hot sauce.

Another popular condiment is salsa, which is a tomato-based sauce that is commonly used in Mexican cuisine. Salsa can be made with fresh or canned tomatoes, and a variety of chillies and spices. To make a basic salsa, you will need to chop tomatoes, onions, and chillies, and then mix them together with lime juice, cilantro, and salt. Salsa can be adjusted to your desired level of heat by using different types of chillies.

Chutneys are also popular condiments that are commonly used in Indian and Southeast Asian cuisine. Chutneys are made by simmering fruits, vegetables, or herbs with chillies, vinegar, and sugar. The mixture is then pureed until smooth and can be served with a variety of dishes. Some popular chutneys include mango chutney, tamarind chutney, and mint chutney.

Pickling is another popular method of preserving chillies. Pickled chillies are commonly used in sandwiches, salads, and as a condiment for meats. To pickle chillies, you will need to mix vinegar, water, salt, and sugar in a pot and bring the mixture to a boil. Add sliced chillies to the mixture and let them cool. The pickled chillies can be stored in jars and will keep for several months.

In conclusion, chilli-based condiments and sauces are versatile additions to many dishes and can be made at home with a few simple ingredients. Whether you prefer hot sauce, salsa, chutney, or pickled chillies, there are many different recipes and variations to choose from. Experiment with different types of chillies and ingredients to create your own signature sauce or condiment that will add a fiery kick to your favorite meals.

Home Remedies and Traditional Uses of Chillies in Different Cultures

Chillies have been used for their medicinal properties for centuries in various cultures around the world. From alleviating pain to improving digestion, chillies have a wide range of health benefits. In this chapter, we will explore some of the traditional uses and home remedies of chillies in different cultures.

Ayurvedic Medicine: In Ayurvedic medicine, chillies are believed to have a heating effect on the body, which can help stimulate digestion and improve circulation. Chillies are often used in remedies for coughs, colds, and sore throats. One common remedy involves mixing ground chillies with honey to create a paste that can be applied to the throat to alleviate pain.

Traditional Chinese Medicine: In Traditional Chinese Medicine, chillies are believed to have a warming effect on the body, which can help improve blood circulation and stimulate the metabolism. Chillies are often used in remedies for joint pain, arthritis, and muscle soreness. One popular remedy involves steeping chillies in hot water to create a tea that can be consumed to relieve pain.

Mexican Folk Medicine: In Mexican folk medicine, chillies are believed to have a range of healing properties, including the ability to alleviate pain, reduce inflammation, and improve digestion. Chillies are often used in remedies for headaches, arthritis, and stomach issues. One common remedy involves mixing ground chillies with salt and applying the paste to the temples to alleviate headaches.

Indian Ayurveda: In Indian Ayurveda, chillies are believed to have a range of health benefits, including the ability to improve digestion, stimulate circulation, and alleviate pain. Chillies are often used in remedies for colds, coughs, and sore throats. One popular remedy involves mixing ground chillies with turmeric and honey to create a paste that can be applied to the throat to relieve pain.

Caribbean Folk Medicine: In Caribbean folk medicine, chillies are believed to have a range of medicinal properties, including the ability to reduce inflammation, alleviate pain, and improve digestion. Chillies are often used in remedies for joint pain, arthritis, and stomach issues. One common remedy involves steeping chillies in hot water to create a tea that can be consumed to relieve pain.

In conclusion, chillies have been used for their medicinal properties for centuries in different cultures around the world. From alleviating pain to improving digestion, chillies have a wide range of health benefits. While these remedies may not replace conventional medicine, they can be a helpful addition to a healthy lifestyle. As with any natural remedy, it is important to consult with a healthcare professional before using chillies for medicinal purposes.

Chilli Festivals and Competitions: A Celebration of Spice

Chilli festivals and competitions are becoming increasingly popular around the world, drawing in thousands of visitors who share a love for all things spicy. These events are a celebration of the diversity and versatility of chillies, showcasing the various varieties, cuisines, and cultures that incorporate them into their cuisine. In this chapter, we will explore some of the most notable chilli festivals and competitions around the world and the unique experiences they offer.

One of the largest chilli festivals in the United States is the National Fiery Foods and Barbecue Show, held annually in Albuquerque, New Mexico. This three-day event brings together over 200 exhibitors and features spicy food tastings, cooking demonstrations, and live entertainment. Visitors can sample a wide range of spicy foods and sauces, including some of the hottest chillies in the world. The event also includes a chili cook-off competition, where participants compete for the title of best chili recipe.

In Australia, the annual Hottest 100 Chilli Festival is held in Geelong, Victoria. This event showcases some of the hottest chillies grown in Australia and features a range of activities, including cooking demonstrations, live music, and a chilli-eating competition. The festival also includes a marketplace where visitors can purchase chilli products and fresh produce.

In the United Kingdom, the Great Dorset Chilli Festival is a popular event held in the county of Dorset. This two-day festival features over 140 stalls selling chilli-related products, including sauces, dips, and spices. Visitors can sample a wide range of international cuisine, attend cooking demonstrations, and take part in chilli-eating challenges.

In Thailand, the Nong Khai Chilli Festival is a well-known event that celebrates the country's love for spicy food. Held annually in Nong Khai province, the festival features a range of chilli-related activities, including cooking competitions, chilli-eating challenges, and cultural performances. Visitors can also purchase a variety of chilli products and fresh produce from local vendors.

Other notable chilli festivals and competitions include the International Hot and Spicy Food Festival in Ontario, Canada, the Bowers Chile Pepper Festival in Pennsylvania, USA, and the Harissa Festival in Nabeul, Tunisia.

In conclusion, chilli festivals and competitions offer a unique opportunity to celebrate the diverse and flavorful world of spicy food. Whether you are a seasoned chilli aficionado or a newcomer to the world of heat, these events offer a fun and exciting way to experience the many different varieties and cultures that incorporate chillies into their cuisine.

Conclusion: A Spicy World of Flavor and Health

In conclusion, chillies have long been a staple in kitchens around the world, prized for their ability to add flavor, heat, and health benefits to a variety of dishes. From the mild jalapeno to the fiery ghost pepper, there is a chili variety to suit every taste and culinary need.

Through the course of this book, we have explored the many facets of chillies, from their cultivation and harvesting to their use in a variety of cuisines and condiments. We have delved into the science of heat, understanding Scoville units and capsaicin content, and learned how to pair different chili varieties with ingredients to create delicious and balanced flavor profiles.

We have also looked at the traditional and home remedies uses of chillies in different cultures and how they are celebrated in festivals and competitions around the world. Through it all, we have discovered the versatility, complexity, and beauty of this small but mighty ingredient.

Whether you are a seasoned chili enthusiast or a curious beginner, there is always more to learn and explore in the world of chillies. So go forth, experiment, and savor the endless possibilities that this spicy world has to offer.

Scoville scale

The Scoville scale is a measurement of the spicy heat or pungency of chili peppers and other spicy foods. It was named after American pharmacist Wilbur Scoville, who developed the scale in 1912. The scale is based on the concentration of capsaicin, the compound responsible for the spiciness of chili peppers. The scale ranges from 0 (no heat) to over 2 million Scoville heat units (SHU) for the spiciest peppers in the world, such as the Carolina Reaper and the Trinidad Moruga Scorpion. The Scoville scale is commonly used in the food industry to indicate the spiciness of different products, from mild to extremely hot.

Scoville Heat Units (SHU)	Spiciness Level	Examples
0-100	No heat	Bell peppers, sweet peppers
100-500	Mild	Poblano peppers, banana peppers
500-2,500	Medium	Jalapeño peppers, chipotle peppers
2,500-8,000	Hot	Serrano peppers, Tabasco sauce
8,000-50,000	Very hot	Cayenne pepper, Sriracha sauce

50,000-100,000	Extremely hot	Habanero peppers, Scotch bonnet peppers
100,000-350,000	Dangerously hot	Ghost peppers, Trinidad Scorpion pepper
350,000-2,200,000	World's hottest	Carolina Reaper, Pepper X

Note that these ranges are approximate and can vary depending on the specific variety of chili pepper and how it is grown, harvested, and prepared. Also, individual tolerance to spiciness can vary widely, so what one person considers mild may be too hot for another.

Other books by the author

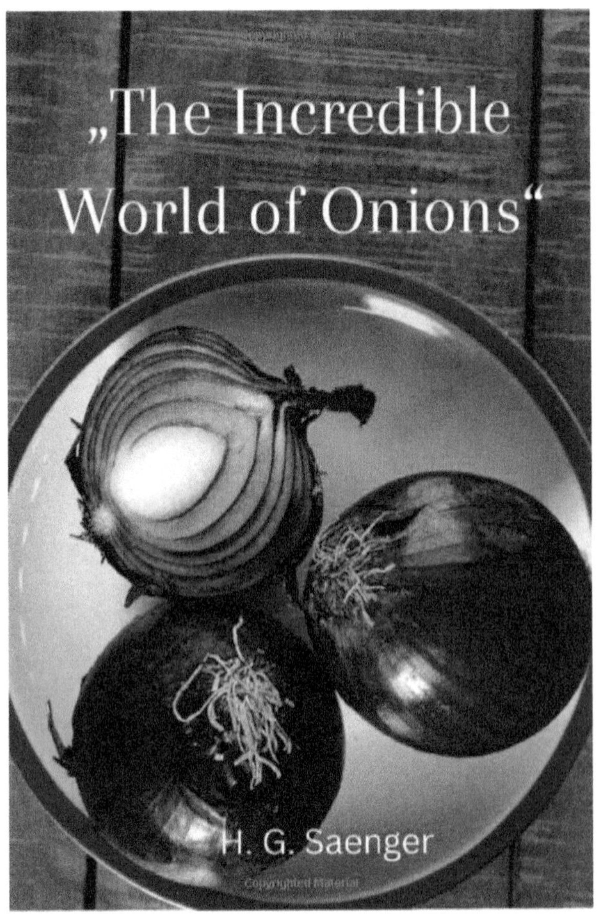

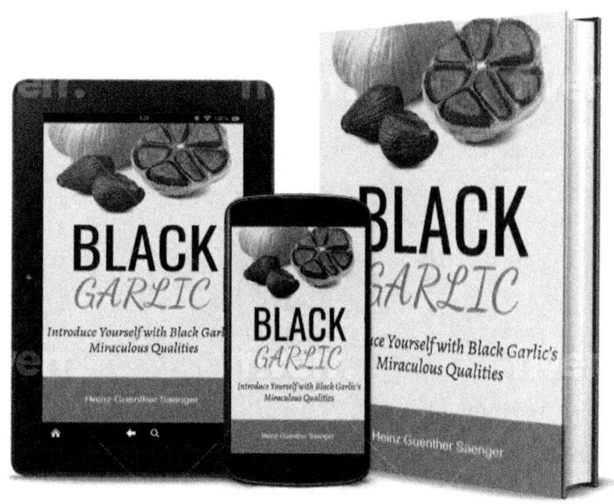
BLACK
GARLIC
Introduce Yourself with Black Garlic's
Miraculous Qualities
Heinz Guenther Saenger

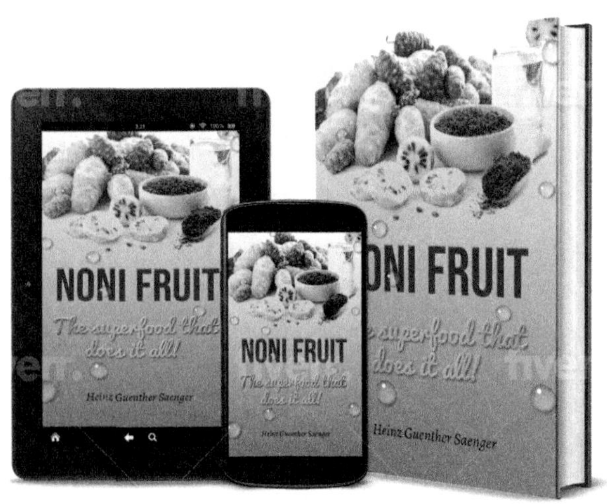
NONI FRUIT
The superfood that does it all!
Heinz Guenther Saenger

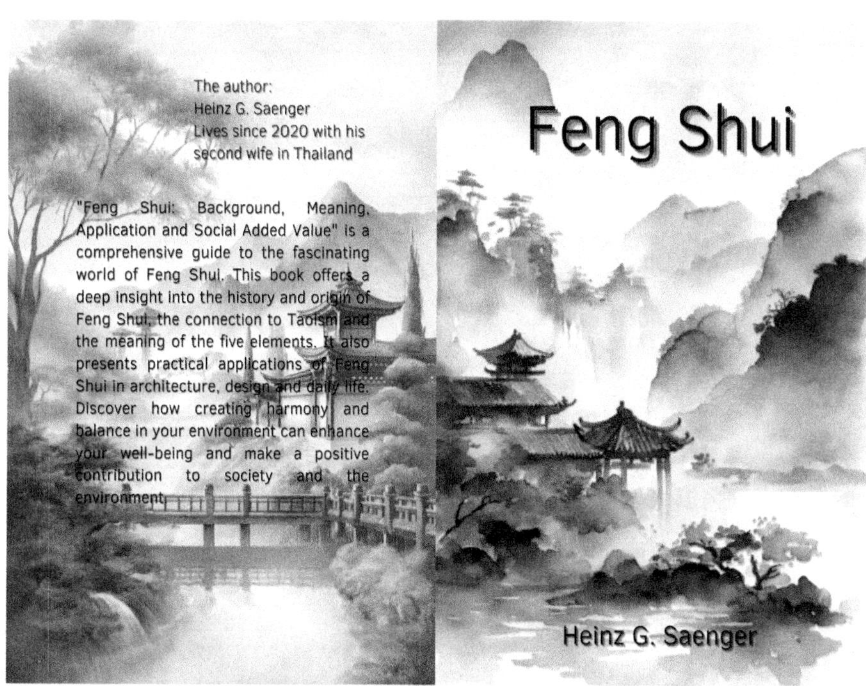
The author:
Heinz G. Saenger
Lives since 2020 with his second wife in Thailand
"Feng Shui: Background, Meaning, Application and Social Added Value" is a comprehensive guide to the fascinating world of Feng Shui. This book offers a deep insight into the history and origin of Feng Shui, the connection to Taoism and the meaning of the five elements. It also presents practical applications of Feng Shui in architecture, design and daily life. Discover how creating harmony and balance in your environment can enhance your well-being and make a positive contribution to society and the environment.
Feng Shui
Heinz G. Saenger

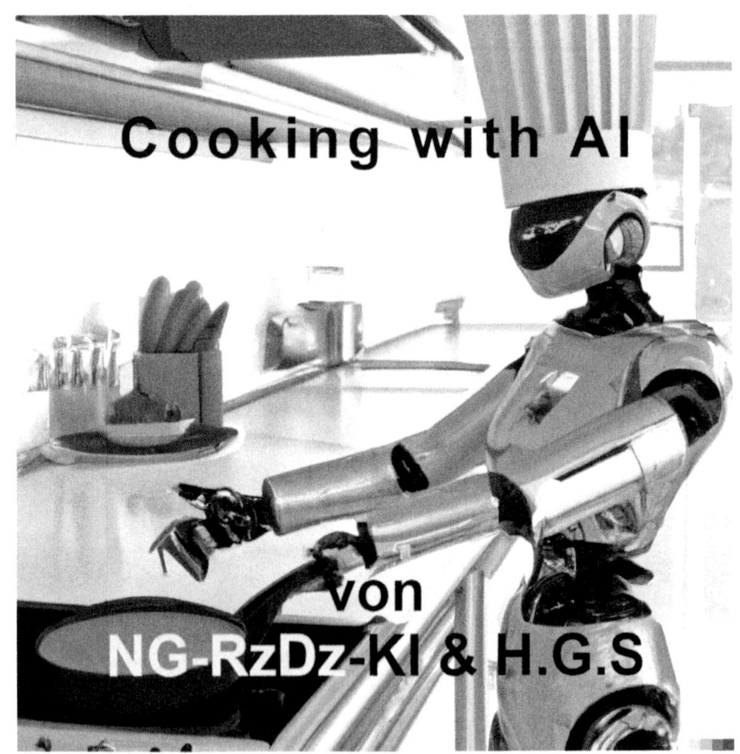
Cooking with AI
von
NG-RzDz-KI & H.G.S

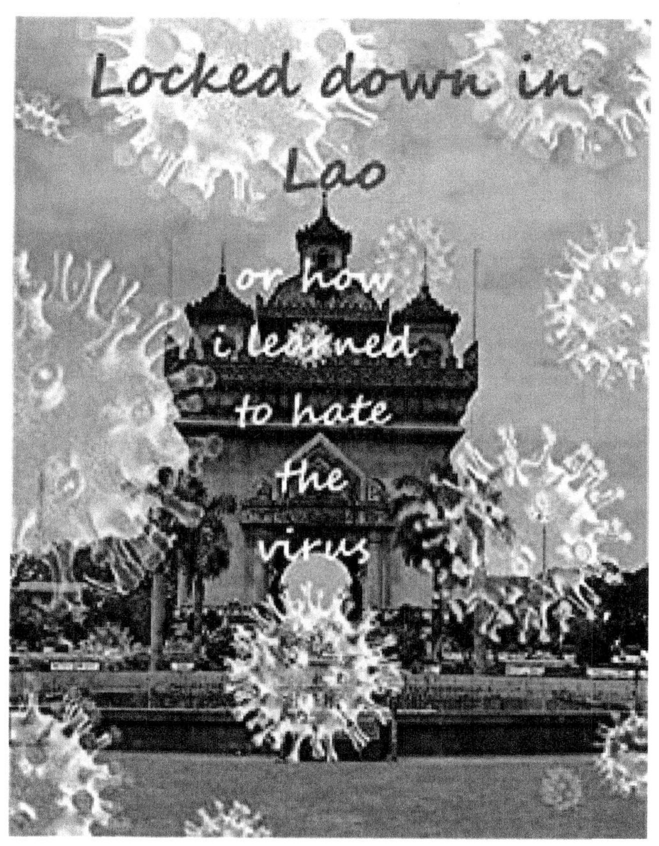
Locked down in
Lao
or how
i learned
to hate
the
virus

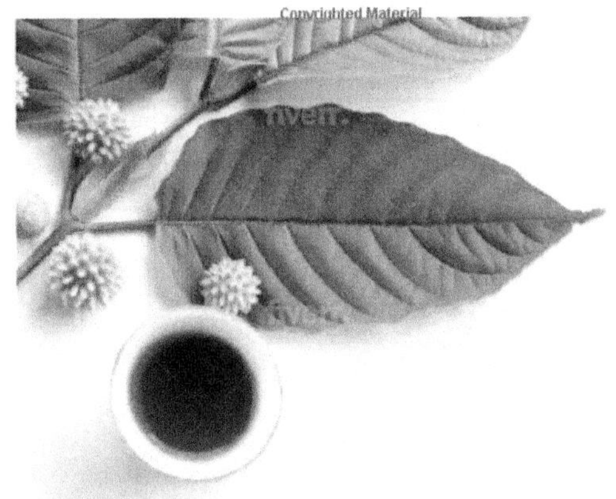

KRATOM FOR NEWBIES

All You Need To Know About Kratom Usage

By Heinz Guenther Saenger

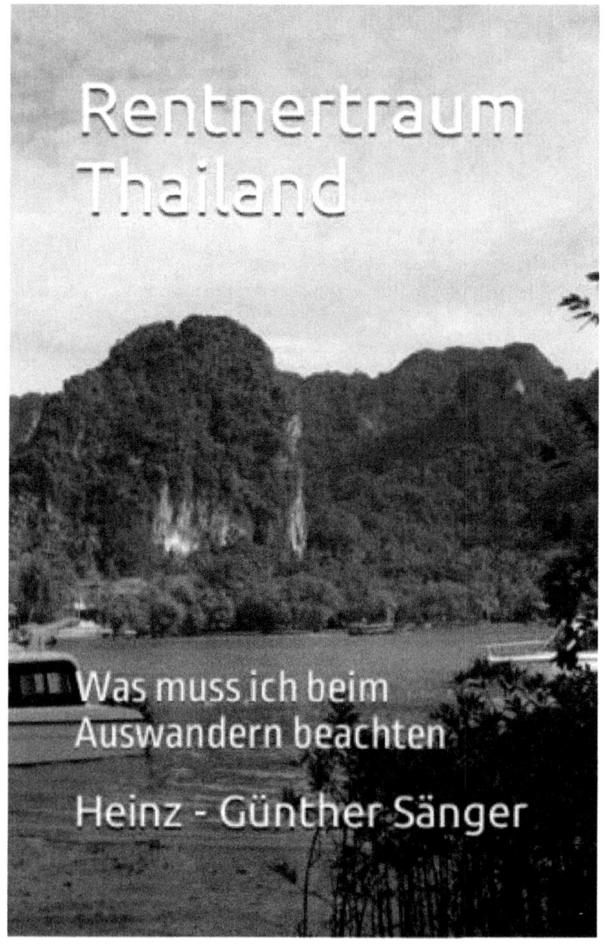
Rentnertraum
Thailand
Was muss ich beim
Auswandern beachten
Heinz - Günther Sänger

Printed in Great Britain
by Amazon

27447016R00046